Body Integration

& The One Minute Workout

Learning to Love the Body You're In
Version 2.4

By: Michael Morris Phoenix

Copyright Notice:

© 2019 – Michael J.M. Phoenix - All Rights Reserved.

All rights reserved. No part of this publication may be reproduced, distributed, or transmitted in any form or by any means, including photocopying, recording, or other electronic or mechanical methods, without the prior written permission of the publisher, except in the case of brief quotations embodied in critical reviews and certain other noncommercial uses permitted by copyright law. For permission requests, write to the publisher, addressed "Attention: Permissions Coordinator," at the address below.

Emergent Strategies LLC
PO Box 245
Winona, MO. 65588
https://3m3r3g.com
orders@3m3rg3.com

Ordering Information:

ISBN: 978-1-7337454-3-7

Quantity sales. Special discounts are available on quantity purchases by corporations, associations, and others. For details, contact the publisher at the address above.

For more in-depth instruction on this method Body Integration visit https://MichaelPhoenix.Me.

Cover Art: Sam Whelan https:SamWhelan.net

Change Log

Version 1.0 – 20130415: Initial Draft.

Version 1.1 – 20160220: Minor revisions to wording throughout.

Version 1.2 – 20161015: Updates to Phase 1, Sections 1, 2, 3, 4. Initial draft of Phase 1, Sections 5, 6.

Version 2.0 – 20170101: Major edit of Phase 1, Sections 3, 4, 5.

Version 2.1 – 20180228: Minor phrase revisions throughout the Orientation. Initial draft of Phase 2.

Version 2.2 – 20180931: Minor revisions throughout. Preface added. Further development of Phase 2.

Version 2.3 – 20190209: Further development of Phase 2.

Version 2.4 – 20190711: Minor revisions or grammar and formatting.

Contents

Change Log 2
It All Begins Somewhere 6
Body Integration | Mode Zero: Finding the Balance 12
    Section 1: Breath Awareness 12
        1.1 – In 13
        1.2 – Out 14
    Section 2: Bone Awareness 15
        2.1 – Structure 16
        2.2 – Balance 16
    Section 3: Muscle Awareness 17
        3.1 – Contract 17
        3.2 – Relax 18
    Section 4: Joint Awareness 19
        4.1 – Range 20
        4.2 – Motion 20
    Section 5: Sense Awareness 22
        5.1 - Felt Experience 23
        5.2 - Attention Point 24
        5.3 - Proprioception 24
Body Integration | Phase 1: The One Minute Workout 27
    Section 1: Core Focus 27
        1.1 - Coccyx 28
        1.2 – Perineum 28
        1.3 – Abdominals 28
        1.4 - Back Extensors 29

    1.5 - Oblique's 29

  Section 2: Contraction 29

  Section 3: Relaxation 32

  Section 4: Stretching 33

  Section 5: Recovery 34

  Section 6: Integration 35

Body Integration | Phase 2: Learning to Love the Body You're In 37

  Section 1: Emotional Resilience....................................37

  Section 2: Facing the Pain...38

    2.1 Inflammation 39

    2.2 Relaxed Shoulders and Hips...............................40

    2.3 Stabilized Feet...40

    2.4 Supple Jaw 42

    2.5 Sensitive Hands..42

  Section 3: Breath Integrity..43

    3.1 Guiding the Breath...44

    3.2 Breathing Open the Shoulders and Hips..........47

    3.3 Breathing Into the Feet.....................................48

    3.4 Breathing Down the Jaw 49

    3.5 Breathing Through the Palms 49

  Section 4: Posture Equilibrium 50

    4.1 Posture of the Hips 52

    4.2 Posture of the Shoulders 53

    4.3 Posture of the Feet 54

    4.4 Posture of the Hands 55

    4.5 Posture of the Jaw 56

Section 5: Tension Analysis and Release 58

    5.1 Shoulder Analysis and Release 60

    5.2 Hip Analysis and Release 61

    5.3 Foot Analysis and Release 62

    5.4 Jaw Analysis and Release 62

    5.5 Hand Analysis and Release 63

Section 6: Emotional Integrity 63

Section 7: Paradigm of Integrity 65

Section 8: Eliminating Waste 66

Section 9: Additional One Minute Workouts 67

    9.1 Seated Gluteus Wave 68

    9.2 Standing Gluteus Wave 68

    9.2 For More, Go Here 69

Other Titles and Works by Michael Phoenix 70

It All Begins Somewhere

In my case, it was something my mom said about me as a child.

She says I used to always be a happy kid. A care-free spirit.

Then something changed. It was like I lost that spark and she didn't know why.

The reality is, no one knew why. It took me 19 years to remember. I was a 27 year old newly-wed, two months into my marriage with a woman whom I adored. My dream-come-true, literally.

I was 9 when I had a dream about my wedding day. It was one of two moments in my childhood that I can tell you, without question, I felt the emotion of happiness. A dream.

In fact, both those moments where I remember feeling happy, were dreams. The other dream was a few years later. I can't point to any actual life experiences where I felt pure happiness. Only two dreams.

So when I started to remember the childhood sexual abuse that I was victim to, and subsequently began destroying my dream-come-true because I had no emotional process to deal with what was happening, it was this theory, and a whole lot of counseling, that has given me freedom in my emotions. Not freedom *from* my emotions. But a freedom to actually feel the fullness of **all** my emotions. Without fear of what I may do with them.

Freedom!

I had always been passionate about fitness. Since 7th grade when I started training for football with two of my 5 older brothers. We we're all starting new journeys in our football careers. Pat, his first year of college football after a phenomenal high school career. John, his first year of high school football. And me, as a 7th grader in my first year of organized football. "Focused" would be the

Body Integration

word I'd use to describe us 3 back then. "Determined" may be another.

This theory began about that same time when I realized that I enjoyed stretching. I was around 13.

Some people may enjoy running, or riding bikes. I enjoyed stretching. So, I had an idea. Teach myself how to stretch really well. Be the world's best stretcher. Maybe not the most flexible, but definitely the best at doing exactly what my body needed to feel good. I also wanted to be a quarterback in the NFL. Some dreams just aren't meant to be ;)

Anyway, over time that idea has evolved into this theory. So when I started to realize that, as a 27 year old man, with 4 children, a wife, and the emotional range of a gnat and no emotional process to speak of, I figured I better get busy figuring something out. It took 8 years and me destroying my marriage to get it figured out, but I can tell you, without doubt, I'm happier and healthier than I've ever been.

I actually love being alive now. And feel joy regularly.

I no longer need to meditate for hours to get to that space of joy either. With a few breaths, in almost any situation, joy is immediately available.

This is a far cry from my emotional experience growing up – calmness 75% of the time, anger and rage the other 25%. Violent rage in fact. And if you're curious to get a glimpse what that looked like in the form of my 17-year-old self, I invite you to preview on Amazon the first chapter of my book "Facing Revelation: An Emerging".

This theory all came together one night, 13 days after my 28th solar return (birthday), March 5th, 2011. Standing in my living room at 2AM, unable to sleep. Reflecting on having just cremated my son's 4-month-old dog after I had inadvertently run it over that morning. The guilt in my stomach, and shame in my chest waked back and forth as waves in the ocean. The anger beginning to course through me as a narrative of being a horrible father snared my mind in a back-and-forth debate with myself.

High from a few good-sized micro-doses of a fat joint, clarity began to emerge. A sense of knowing that I needed to do something to exert a whole lot of energy, I started a muscle-contraction technique I came up with a few years previous.

Starting in my core, and with every breath I would flex a single muscle to the tightest contraction I could. From the perineum up to the top of the chest. With each new breath, I'd add a new region of my body, integrating a new muscle to the process. Leaving my arms, legs, and head relaxed.

My intent in that moment was to burn the anger away. Fight fire with fire. And I was determined to not "let it out" except through exercise. As I released the intensity of that contraction, my body washed over with relaxation. I immediately moved to the floor and began stretching.

As I lay on the floor, it was the surge of sensation in my tailbone that took my breath away. It was the first time that I felt the depth of anger. Before that, anger had always felt like flames burning from the inside out, in my chest, arms, and legs.

This anger was different. It felt like molten lava just below my solar plexus. An urge to spew it out on the world around me began forming in my stomach. I swallowed a deep gulp of air into my stomach.

A sharp pain in my lower back began to present itself. I inhaled a deep breath and moved into happy-baby pose. As my hands pressed my feet deeper into the pose, a memory of my 8-year-old-self flashed across my mind. A dullness washed through my chest as I witnessed the memory show me an older boy do what

Body Integration

he pleased with me. His mom looking on with twisted delight next to us on the bed.

My stomach began to clench tight as my mind's eye narrowed to my hands in the memory. Grasping my ankles in similar fashion to happy baby pose, I felt myself lift from my body as if I was no longer in it. Floating by a nearby window, I saw the boy continuing to do what he pleased.

Taken aback, I snapped my mind away from the memory and my put attention-point on feeling the sensation of inhaling air into my lungs. I eased the pressure off the soles of my feet and relaxed my diaphragm. Lifting my chest, I moved my body to create a vacuum pressure in the chest cavity. Gently pulling air in through my nose, and down into my abdomen. Slowly inhaling to a full breath, I moved the tips of my fingers to the tips of my toes. My thumbs gently pressing on the tops of my big toes.

With full breath, I put my consciousness back into my 8-year-old self and allowed my 27-year-old self to feel the fullness of that experience. A rush of emotion and sensation flushed through me. Sadness, pleasure, disgust, anger, curiosity, confusion. Laying there on the floor, allowing my mind to play through the scene, my body began to move through the motions of the memory.

Over the course of the next two hours, I purposefully followed the winding narrative of these memories as they arose. I would follow the journey of my body movements, replaying them. Holding the specific intent to finally allow myself a processing of the experience. Giving my body over to my breath every step of the way.

Before that night of surging sensation in my tailbone, breath work had already been a central aspect of my overall mindfulness practice. After that night, however, it became a primary focus for understanding the power of emotion in my body. The more skilled I became at breathing, the more internal space I was able to

Body Integration

create for the process of recovering from the emotional trauma of childhood sexual abuse.

What follows in this book, is my best attempt at articulating 3 different aspects of this theory. 1) A mental frame as a premise. 2) A context of what to focus on in the core (thoracic region) while conducting experiments with this theory. And lastly, certain areas of exploration for further refinement to embody this as a daily practice.

As a practice, it is understood that if you choose to begin experimenting, you do so at the accountability of your own free will. What's given here is only information. What you do with this information is entirely up to you. Seek professional counsel if you're unsure about your path forward.

When asked what "body integration" is, I summarize it as a synthesis of yoga, tai chi, and exercise physiology. That said, I'm not a certified yoga teacher, nor am I a tai chi master, and I don't have a degree in exercise physiology. What I am, however, is an intelligent, compassionate man in this world, using the fullness of his capacities to not only recover from intense childhood trauma, but thrive in a state of sustaining joy.

To that end, as I've journeyed through life, I've picked up a lot of jewels from a lot of different places. Starting with athletics in high school and college, to military physical fitness, to yoga retreats, tai chi classes, counseling/therapy/mentoring of many different kinds, to plain old health and exercise science.

In my life, that idea I had as 13-year-old has seen me through many trials and tribulations. From needing to stabilize my core to cope with a career ending (football) condition in my L5 vertebra called spondylolistheses, to the emotional and sensatory processing by way of recovering from childhood sexual abuse, to most recently recovering from reconstructive surgery in my left ankle, right knee, left elbow, as well as fluid in my left lung after it collapsed due to a near fatal motorcycle accident.

As I live my life, I will not accept a diminished quality of life. I enjoy playing basketball, riding horses, hiking, swimming, as well as many other things that require me to be healthy in mind, body, and soul. The purpose of this theory is to help others achieve this same space – enjoying life.

That said, this is a living practice. Emotional integrity in synergy with a functional proficiency in body movement is the specific goal. There is no final-destination to seek, but rather an enjoyment of the process of being human.

There is a richness that can be found, simply by giving yourself the opportunity to resolve any residual suffering that may be in the body. In this, listening to the body, as a curious student would to a master teacher, is what facilitates this integration. The practicing is not about trying to find the ideal of perfection in the form of a yoga pose, or precision of a tai chi movement. This is a practice of becoming ever mindful of the sense of release that occurs in your body as you listen to the subtle movements it needs for the tension to release *permanently*.

Mastery of this doesn't happen overnight. This movement, to integrate the fullness of your human experience, is a life-long journey. No matter what your specific trauma may be, it is my hope that what's contained herein benefits your ability to stabilize joy in your life.

Body Integration | Mode Zero: Finding the Balance

"I trust that my body knows what to do..."

Section 1: Breath Awareness

The more breath awareness is integrated as living practice, the more the body creates a space for health to reside. Allowing your lungs to teach you how to breathe is a life-long journey with fundamental changes to your-way-life. Body Integration, as a methodology, represents a shift of paradigms.

Body Integration is not something extra that you do when the time is right. Integrating the body is like your breath. It's always happening.

You're either facilitating the process as an active participant in the expression of wisdom, or you're a passive observer letting your health go in the direction of your habits. The question is whether you're okay with letting your health be the result of your habits, or if you desire a change of direction for yourself. Only you know the answer to that question.

Becoming aware of your breath and allowing your lungs to be the guide toward full functional capacity has the consequence of shifting your paradigms. The choice is not if integrating the breath will or will not shift your paradigm, the choice is to let your breath teach you. If you do not make *Breath* Integration the single most important feature of your life, *Body* Integration will remain as something else you have on your to do list.

This is a choice only you can make, and you must come to understand the imperative nature of this choice by direct experience. It is a pill you must pick up and swallow for it to show you what you want to know.

Body Integration

The bottom line is, breathing happens. If it didn't, you're body dies. Refining your skill of breathing is refining your skill in being human.

In Breath Awareness, there is the reality that no other person on this planet can show you how to do it. The same is true with Body Integration. And that is why this is presented as a theory. Because for you, it is theory. It may be a fact for me, but it has only become so through application of what's presented here.

Becoming a student of Your lungs will shape your mind and prepare you to be a student of your body. Being a student of your body helps to connect a certain type of circuitry that exists at a causal basis of the state of health you are seeking.

Allow your lungs to show you how to breathe a full breath. Allow your lungs to show you how to integrate breathing full breaths on a regular basis. As you become more aware of what your lungs are guiding you toward, the more you are integrating breath awareness.

1.1 – In

The lungs are composed of tiny sacs called alveoli. In these sacs is an alveolar membrane. And through the process of diffusion, carbon dioxide moves out of the blood, and oxygen moves in. You experience this daily, with every breath.

As breathing happens, not all the sacs release old air and bring in new air. As you yawn, your lungs force open all the alveoli for a maximum exchange of air. Your VO2 max is the maximum amount of oxygen that can be brought in during the process of breathing. The higher the VO2 max, the quicker your recovery. In terms of an athlete, say a wide receiver in football, being able to run routes on a consecutive basis is fundamentally tied to his ability to recover. His breathing ability is the foundation of this recover-ability. The same is true for any athlete.

Body Integration

Breathing with shallow breaths engages a minimized functional lung capacity. Breathing full breaths engages a maximized functional capacity. Breathing full breaths is contingent upon how much air you can bring to your lungs with each breath, as well as the rate of exchange of carbon dioxide and oxygen. The higher the exchange rate with each breath, the more oxygen your blood gets.

Oxygen is a purifier of the body. It cleans your blood. It provides energy for the cells. It keeps things going.

Through the simple act of taking full breaths, you can begin to reshape your body. If you can teach yourself to yawn with any breath, you will have reached a pinnacle of breath integration. From that point, you must learn to fly. And to do this you must bring the degree of breath awareness into the rest of your body's systems.

1.2 – Out

As you breathe out or exhale, you get to let go of control. As you let go of control, you get to witness the experience of enjoying fresh oxygen circulate through your body. You know this feeling most often when you yawn. In a yawn, your body is trying to tell you something – wake up!

We often associate a yawn with being tired. In reality, yawning often emerges from a build-up of stagnant energy – old air as one aspect of that energy. And as you yawn, your body is flushing that energy out. Notice that a wide-open mouth with stretched jaw muscles is indicative of a yawn.

If you release your jaw and open it wide, as if you are yawning, you may actually induce a yawn. Try this now. If a yawn occurs, notice the function of air intake as a process. Don't attempt to control the air intake. Simply let the intake process occur and

Body Integration

observe it from a neutral point of view as a scientist observing an experiment.

Also notice that the body's initial reaction on waking up in the morning is to stretch and take deep, full breaths. Watch a young child as she awakens. You will notice this quite often. When you wake up in the morning, notice the sensation in your body. Is it asking you to stretch? Is it asking you to take a deep breath? Notice if my suggestion is planting a seed for your awareness, or if Your body actually WANTS to stretch and breathe deeply, irrespective of my suggestion. Be as unbiased as you can as you observe and witness the body's sensatory mechanisms.

Section 2: Bone Awareness

Sensing the posture of your body allows you to gauge the balance of the structure of your body. From a perspective of 'systems analysis', the bones are the foundation upon which your ability *to do* finds its locomotive basis. Anybody who has experienced a sprained ankle understands the imperative nature of proper bone alignment.

The same is true for all joints of the body. Have you ever jammed a finger? This occurs through a force being exerted on the system in such a way wherein the force exerts pressure in directions the bones were not meant to go. Aligning the bone structure of the body is inherently linked to the joints and joint awareness.

Begin by noticing all the ways in which your posture is out of proper alignment. "Proper alignment" is defined as a symmetry in the balance of the bones that is unique to your bone anatomy.

No two bodies are the same. There are similarities. But your bones are yours. You sensing into the intimacy of this principle will cultivate the space required to feel into the alignment of your bones. See proper balance in your mind's eye and gauge if the sensations in your body synthesizes with the sense of balance established by the image in your mind. Stand in front of a mirror and notice your posture. Experiment with what feels balanced in yourself.

In doing this, you will need to be sure that you are not finding a point in which you find relief but is still actually out of balance. This point of relief may be part of the journey, but is still not proper balance. It requires diligence to undo years of the same unbalanced posture.

2.1 – Structure

Bones are the foundation. Muscles are attached to bones by way of tendons. Ligaments hold bones together at the joints. As any landscaper knows, the first row of blocks in a retaining wall is the most important. If a block is off by even the slightest of measurements, it translates through the rest of the wall. And by the time you get to the top, the half-inch can become half a foot depending on the size of the wall.

The same is true for your bones. If the skull is not properly aligned on the spine, no matter what you do to the rest of your spine to find alignment, it will never reach full alignment and will eventually fall out of alignment. Your head leads. Where you head goes, your body follows. Said another way, you managing your attention point is of utmost priority. Your point of focus determines to a large extent the result that is your quality of life.

2.2 – Balance

Balance is alignment. A symptom of being out of alignment is a sensation of pain at transition points, or joints. To find balance, and integrate it, the muscles are used to pull and push the body back into its proper posture. And from there, contracting the muscles toward a muscle memory of proper posture is the way of Body Integration.

As you find balance, you may notice a greater awareness of all the ways the body is out of alignment. No worries. The joy of Body Integration is that you simply continue moving forward in small steps. The journey is long, the steps are small.

Section 3: Muscle Awareness

The more you are aware of your body, the more you can direct it toward your passions. Having a greater potential *to do work* is inherently linked to your muscular control. As you type on the keyboard, it's the muscles that are moving your fingers.

The theory of Body Integration states that if there is excessive fat build up in a certain area of the body, the one who owns that body is not consciously using the muscles to function in their fullest capacity. More specifically, the muscles come nowhere near reaching their fullest functional capacity.

A dormant muscle is a muscle that becomes weak. In some this presents as being skinny and atrophied (this is my body type). In others, weakness can present as a build up of fat. In either case, the weakness of the muscle is due to a lack of conscious engagement of that muscle.

There are muscles in your body right now that you are not aware of. If you tried to flex that muscle with proprioception, you could not do it.

Test this, find a weak area of your body and try to individually flex the muscles of that area. You might start that exploration with your inner thigh.

3.1 – Contract

A contraction occurs as a neural signal is passed by way of the brain, through the nerves, to the receptors in the muscle. A lightning flash of neurons blast when a muscle is contracting. Taking a contraction to its maximal flex is a key focus.

Body Integration

Integration contraction occurs by engaging each muscle fiber proprioceptively in progressions of intensity toward maximal capacity. In doing this, movement of the body becomes a conscious activity.

Muscle contraction is force-positive. As you increase the awareness of your muscles moving through ranges of motion, and integrate that awareness into a zone of focus for the whole body toward accomplishing purpose, the more you have integrated your body to be a vessel through which you can achieve the dreams in your life.

Your ability *to do work* is inherently linked to your ability to move muscles, too include the brain. Intellectual understanding of this material is one thing. Operational understanding is something altogether different.

3.2 – Relax

Relaxing a muscle occurs naturally. It represents your release of control. Much of the rhetoric of this theory talks about being "in control." And yet, your ability to release control is just as instrumental to your overall ability to do work, if not more important.

If you did not release your breath, you'd eventually pass out, at which point the release would happen automatically. Moreover, releasing the waste from the lungs is the only way fresh air can come in. The release is natural. You have no control over what happens after the release, only the mechanism of the releasing function.

Relaxation is a surrender of control. As the theory goes, integrating a deeper level of awareness in the relaxation of your muscles integrates a deeper potential for the appreciation of life. If you've ever *enjoyed* a massage, you understand this aspect of the theory quite well.

Body Integration

Conversely, if you notice a muscle you're unable to relax, it's a muscle that has a memory of tension to a degree that you are unaware of how to surrender control of that tension. The result of this is stress. The stress of habituated tension in the muscle has the effect of stress chemicals constantly being introduced into your body. This degree of dis-ease can lead to many downstream issues. **Identification of habituated tension and integrating relaxation is a primary focus** with regard to reducing stress as a movement toward increasing emotional resilience.

Section 4: Joint Awareness

Without joints, you are as a board, and movement is not possible. Nurturing your joints is crucial to the success of Body Integration. Much stagnant energy finds itself in the joints of the body. For example, when you yawn, your jaw joint is a primary focus of the release of stagnant energy. Notice yourself the next time you yawn. Pay close attention to the sensations of your jaw, neck and upper chest. Also notice the top of your head. And as you become more aware of these sensations, also integrate an awareness of your perineum and the tip of your tailbone as the yawn unfolds. Notice the sensations.

The single action of yawning affects all these areas in significant ways. And this is just one joint. Imagine all the rest of your joints where there is a buildup of energy that can't find its release.

What happens to electricity when it builds in a system past the point of the system's ability to functionally handle the amount of energy? In a house with a breaker box, a breaker will pop for that part of the system.

Notice what happens to electronics during a lightning strike on a house that has not been grounded.

The same is true for the human body. Proper grounding of the circuitry is critical to emotional resilience. Emotional resilience is critical to an overall state of health. As the joints are able to release the static energy (inflammation, rigidity in the ligaments, etc.), the body's circuits approach a greater capacity to harness the bio-electric energies it requires to function.

4.1 – Range

The range of a joint is the state-space that the appendage can move within. The knee is a hinge joint that has a specific range with a single plane of movement. The shoulder is a ball and socket that has a different range with multiple planes of movement.

Each joint's range is unique. Ideally, the range of your left knee should be the same as your right. However, this is most often not the case. Anyone with a knee injury understands this.

Understanding the range of Your joints requires joint awareness. No one else can tell you what your range is, even yourself. Your range as it exists currently, is influenced by your level of fitness that you've integrated into your body as guided by your focal points. For example, the muscular flexibility in each muscle associated to the joint significantly impacts the range of movement.

As you integrate a more functional degree of fitness into the body, you'll integrate a more functional range. The bone structure of the joint is significant factor for the limit of that range. If you take a joint past its natural limit, you will dislocate the joint. It is imperative that you are intimately in-tune with the range of your joints. Coming to know your boundaries, in all ways (mental, emotional, physical, spiritual, relational, financial, etc.), and honoring those boundaries is critical to a healthy state.

4.2 – Motion

As movement occurs, motion is present. As a human, you are always in motion. You have no choice to not be in motion. If you were not in motion, you'd be dead.

Body Integration

That being the case, understanding the motions of your body, and being aware of its motion is critical to integrating the body into a more functional system.

In terms of joints, motion of the body is only possible through joints. The internal systems, such as the heart, are not contingent upon joints for movement. The heart will continue to beat. Yet, to use the full power of the heart towards enjoying life, the motion of the joints is a primary focal point. The joints where the rib cage connects to the sternum has direct impact on the capacity of the heart. A depressed rib cage can be an indicator of a depressed emotional state. A depressed emotional state is an indicator that the function of breathing can be significantly improved. Not only does a full breath expand the rib cage, it also brings equanimity to the mind, elimination of waste in the body, and stability to the emotions. All these factors influence the hearts ability to do its job at optimal capacity. How you hold the posture of the body molds the way the rib cage forms itself around the heart. Proper posture does not come with "sitting up straight". It comes with awareness of integrating stability throughout the thorax.

And again, as with all other systems of Your body, only you can fully integrate the motion of it. Increasing the awareness of the motion of your joints helps to integrate "ways" of moving in the world that are more in tune with the proper balance of all systems.

Take walking for example. Is your walking fluid? Do you put undue stress on certain parts of your body simply by the way you walk? What if you could increase the pleasure of your experience by changing the way you walk?

Check the soles of your favorite pair of shoes. Where are the wear spots? Notice these areas the next time you walk. Is there a certain degree or type of pain/discomfort? What would happen if you switched the motion of your joints even the slightest? Maybe being more exaggerated in your arm swing will bring in a momentum that carries your upper body differently which affects the way your lower legs move, which removes the pressure on that part of your foot. The result of which is a diminished level of pain. Be a scientist and conduct an experiment with how you move yourself in the world.

Your level of awareness, in the motions of your body, allows you to listen to what your body is saying. As you integrate this wisdom, the pleasure of your body is maximized. According to this theory, the human body naturally desires to maximize pleasure. **Increasing pleasure in all the subtle ways compounds the net effect toward *sustainable* joy.**

Section 5: Sense Awareness

All of Body Integration is meaningless without sense awareness. This is the foundation of the practice. *Your* ability to consciously sense *your* body is what distinguishes *your* ability to move into a healthier way of living life.

The awareness of your body occurs as a sensation. A sensation happens by way of an interaction of energy. Whether it's the bio-electric impulse of the heart which causes the heart to pump, or the electro-chemical thought that's firing across the synapses of your brain; your body cannot sense these things unless these basic energies are moving, flowing, and interacting with reality. Your reality.

Only you are in control of your thoughts. You can choose to think certain thoughts. You can motivate yourself to move by many different means of persuasion. Maybe you have tried guilting yourself to workout. Maybe you've been shamed into it by someone else. Maybe you've used sheer will-power to get up and move.

Body Integration

The theory of Body Integration implies that you are gentle with yourself in the persuasions you use to motivate yourself. Due to the fact that Body Integration requires a finely tuned attention to detail, which can only arise through being sensitive with the system, forcing yourself to practice doesn't allow for an unbiased experimentation with this theory. The more you beat the human body, the less it will produce the results you want. The more you nurture the system, the more it will *naturally* desire to do work.

Doing Your work, and **enjoying** it, is the purpose of Body Integration. The work you do is defined by you. You being aware of your body and what your body needs will allow you to define what work is done.

5.1 - Felt Experience

All feelings, whether emotional or sensatory, occur as an experiential reality in the body. We are not trying to interpret what the body is saying, we are simply listening to the body tell us what it knows. It does this through the felt experience.

The more in-touch you can become with your feelings, the more in-touch you can become with your health. The energy of feelings happens in the same body that you use to live life. If these feelings are not processed, they are stored somewhere in the cellular structures of the body. As these energies persist, they become breeding grounds for dis-ease.

Imagine, as a stagnant farm pond, the feelings you have felt over your past that are still locked inside your body. All the scum, bugs, germs, and other outgrowths can only grow out-of-control because of the stagnancy.

Stagnant water is synonymous with filth. Running water is synonymous with purity.

The same is true for the energies of the body. This is not a matter of "right" feelings vs. "wrong" feelings. This metaphor is intended

Body Integration

to point out that unprocessed emotion and pain can become a breeding grounds for disease.

5.2 - Attention Point

Where your attention point goes, your body follows.

What you focus on is what you attract into your reality. If you feel a certain pain in the body and you become negative and begin to pity yourself, this is the emotional thought energy You are inputting into the system. This emotional thought energy translates as negative emotions. The hormones and stress chemicals of these negative emotions break down the integrity of your body's systems. They are negative insofar as they are disharmonious to your experience. The emotion itself is neither "right" nor "wrong". The emotion is only a result that occurs in the body. The causal factor of that emotion is a paradigm you're holding to some degree.

Emotional processing, as an active process in the cognizance of your attention point, is neither wrong, nor bad. Stigmatizing the fact that emotional processing does not occur in logical progressions is a movement away from the power intrinsic to emotions. Paradigms that allow for evolution of thought and are inclusive of ways that may be foreign to your current process, but are still beneficial, are paradigms that move toward growth.

The body, as a unit of movement in the universe, functions best when all systems are harmonious to the other systems. The body relies on the interdependency of systems to move in the existing reality of experience. Managing your attention point is as a gardener tending the garden. What is the garden you're cultivating as your experience in life?

5.3 - Proprioception

There has been a repetition of the way in which The Theory of Body Integration addresses issues. In that, there has been a focus on the way in which certain systems integrate with other systems. The reasoning behind this is based in the dynamic that the human body acts as a system of integrated systems. A clear example of this interdependency of systems is later discussed in the section on Breath Integrity, specifically Diaphragmatic Attenuation. In short, the diaphragm, as a muscle, its fascia, and other connective tissues, impact other systems from the sacroiliac joint in the hips, to the vagus nerve in the head and neck; and a plethora of other systems in between. It is quite literally, the intermediary of proper functioning of the human body. A facilitator of collaboration.

Without the heart, the body dies. Without the head, the body dies. Without the lungs, the body dies. These systems are primary. From that basis, there are other systems that are "system critical". **Proprioceptive awareness of the diaphragm that controls breathing is of a primary focus in Body Integration**. The diaphragm influences these three systems (heart, head, lungs) to a significant extent. Any unresolved inflammation or binding of the fascia of the diaphragm results in dysfunction of the rest of these three systems. Developing an intimate understanding of proprioception is critical to the success of integrating the body.

Proprioception, in general, is the process of becoming ever aware of the individual systems of the body and how they *relate* to the rest of the body. Algebraic thinking comes in handy with this. In terms of Body Integration, proprioception deals primarily with the movement of the joints and becoming aware of the muscles that move the joints individually. Inside of that movement is an awareness that will bring you to face all the ways you hold the emotion of resistance as tension in the body. Unwinding this from your nervous system and **integrating a micro-awareness of joy** into the movements of the body requires a proprioceptive focus in your attention point.

Body Integration

As you begin to test this theory, understand that your ability to proprioceptively tune into your body is where the experimentation occurs. To experiment and test this theory, come to understand proprioception by way of *doing*.

Body Integration | Phase 1: The One Minute Workout

"As I train my mind to remember, I give my body space to heal…"

Section 1: Core Focus

This theory of integrating the body states, "the more the core is balanced and integrated, the healthier your body will be". Central to this theory is proper posture beginning in the spine. There is one pre-condition prior to spine posture, and that is stabilized feet. This will be discussed in Phase 2 of this theory. For now, however, focus on the core as the central pivot point of your entire body. All movement influences or is influenced by the core.

If you wish to turn, you engage your core. If you wish to walk, you engage your core. In fact, if you press down on a surface with your pinky, there are muscles that engage in the forearm, triceps, latissimus dorsi, back extensors, gluteus maximus, and the hamstring. Each of these muscle groups is engaged in the simple movement of applying pressure to the tip of the pinky.

Try it now?

Are you able to sense this?

The key to Body Integration is beginning to sense all parts of your body. The One Minute Workout focuses on the core as the central hub for the purpose of centering yourself into stability. And, this workout can be done literally anywhere, doing anything. All excuses and justifications to the contrary have been purposely factored out of this paradigm. All it requires is **remembering** to invoke the sequence. And there is no better time to remember

Body Integration

than the instant it's recognized that integrating the boy needs to be done.

Stated plainly, this is not something else to put on the "to do" list.

It is something, however, that can be integrated into every aspect of life's movements.

The "core" as defined herein is the coccyx complex (coccygeus, sacrospinous ligament, piriformis, levator ani), the perineum, the abdominals, the back extensors, and both the internal and external obliques.

1.1 - Coccyx

The coccyx, or tailbone, is a generalized focal point. Tuning more deeply into the specificity of proprioceptive awareness, it's the coccygeus, sacrospinous ligament, piriformis, and levator ani that are the micro-nuances of this point. These points in the coccyx region work in tandem with the perineum to bring stability to the root of the spine. Close your mouth, pinch your nose closed, and try to breathe in with a force strong enough to sense the contraction around the coccyx. The muscles sensed are the point of focus. Finding distinction in sensation between all the muscles in this region is a goal of advancing the practice of body integration. There is a new world of sensation available with proprioceptive awareness in this region of the body.

1.2 – Perineum

This is the muscle you can use to stop urination. It is located just in front of the anus. Flex it now and bring all awareness into this muscle as you flex. While doing this, notice any sensation the contraction of the muscle produces in the body.

1.3 – Abdominals

This muscle group, and its connective fascia, extends from tip of the pubic bone up to the bottom of the sternum. I include the

Body Integration

diaphragm and its connective tissue with the abs. The diaphragm is the muscle that controls the flow of air in and out of the lower lungs. The diaphragm is included with the abs to focus a synchronization of abdominal awareness. The more synchronized the breathing is with the core's symmetry of motion, the more integrated movement emerges as a natural state.

1.4 - Back Extensors

Also known as back straps, these muscles are critical in posture. These are the muscles used to bend backward with a hinge point in the lower spine. Lay flat on the ground, face to the floor, and raise your head and shoulders form the ground without using your arms. The muscles used to engage that movement are the back straps.

1.5 - Oblique's

These muscles are on either side of you. From the top of the hip, wrapping around the front to the abs, and around the back to the back extensors, these muscles assist in lateral bending and twisting. Gently pinch the top of your right ear with your right hand. Point your elbow straight out to your side. Now bend sideways trying to touch your elbow to your hip without moving your shoulder or arm. Pivot the movement over the top of the hip bone. The muscles used to engage this movement are the obliques.

Section 2: Contraction

In the context of "body integration", fundamental to muscle contraction is the sense of proprioception. If you need further clarification on what this is, hold out your dominant hand, the one you use to write with, and touch your pinky to your thumb.

Once your thumb and pink are touching, focus only on moving the pinky back to an upright position. Don't let any other fingers

Body Integration

move. Move only the pinky. Now touch it back to the thumb, again, moving only the pinky.

In doing this, you are using only the muscles required to move the pinky. Gaining the "sense" of these individual muscles in relation to the rest of the body is proprioception. And the degree to which you can guide the application of force through these muscles, as well as relax these muscles, is the degree to which you have integrated your body.

Thus, in terms of the One Minute Workout, the goal is to gain an ever-increasing sense of proprioception in the muscles, tendons, ligaments, and joints associated with the core. The method of Body Integration is to take a muscle or muscle group to complete contraction in a conscious extension of will power, and to complete relaxation as a full release of will power (letting go).

And as ability in proprioception grows, the maximal contraction strength grows in direct proportion to the degree of flexibility or elasticity induced by the contract-relax-stretch dynamic. I refer to this as "increasing suppleness". Supple muscular readiness increases the ability to adapt and respond to new situations.

A joint reaches its full range of motion only when the bones in the joint reaches its functional limit. If a muscle is not flexible enough for a joint to freely and comfortably move in a full range of motion, then neither the joint nor the muscle is fully integrated. Thus, the quality of life is diminished. Maximizing both functional contraction and functional flexibility, in the core is a pre-requisite to experiencing body integration.

Stabilizing a solid foundation is only the beginning. Body Integration in full embodiment ventures into multi-layered aspects of an individual's existence. Here in this book, the focus is on establishing the core as the pivot point for a change of basis such that an individual's vector expression can thus coordinate to a new experiential position, or quality of personal experience.

Body Integration

My ability to produce effort in my life directly correlates to the degree to which I have integrated the functional capacities of all the systems that combine to create "me". If you breathe into your abdomen, while engaging the coccyx and the perineum, allowing the abdominals to relax, a state of calm pleasure may arise. From that starting point, in what ways can you make minor movements with your back extensors to open your chest and abdomen further? Then, on exhale, increase the contractive force in the coccyx, and perineum, while releasing contraction of the back extensors, and engaging contraction in the abdominals. Now what micro-movements can you make with the obliques to induce a deeper contraction in the abdominals?

Take the time necessary to isolate an awareness of movement for each muscle. Start with 20% muscular tension as the max contractive force. From there, increase the degree of contraction as you become more aware of each muscle and muscle group. You will know when you reach full muscle contraction, it will start to feel like a cramp. At this point, release the contraction and move into a stretch of the muscle or muscle group while engaging contraction to the symmetrically opposite muscle or muscle group. Moving through a crunch motion to the right will stretch the left back extensor and gluteus. Now reverse the motion. Explore the movement of the core from this perspective throughout the day.

Go Slow!

As each muscle is taken to a deeper conscious-contraction-point, the net result is a greater degree of *functional* strength in the muscle group, as a synergized team of muscles.

The theory of Body Integration arose out of the impetus to increase functional strength through the use of body-weight only. The One Minute Workout is an exercise paradigm designed specifically to increase the functional capacity of the core through a progression toward maximum contraction and relaxation in the muscle groups mentioned above.

Section 3: Relaxation

As the pendulum swings back from contraction, there is relaxation. Test this now. Take a full breath. Intake air into all the alveoli of the lungs, and when you have reached a maximal input of air, let go and relax. Notice that the exhale takes care of itself. The *relaxation* takes care of itself. The only thing you have to do is "let go" of control.

Notice the sensations in your body. No need to interpret these sensations, just notice them. Take another full breath. Then let go. In doing this, you are exercising your diaphragm.

Relaxation of the core is just as imperative as contraction. A muscle will only get stronger through the recovery process. A weight lifter uses weight to add a certain degree of resistance to the muscles. As the muscles resists through the negative movement, small tears occur. As these tears heal, strength and size increase.

Even still, it is possible to reach a plateau. Any athlete has likely encountered this phenomenon. A plateau is indicative of stagnation. And typically, overworking muscles is the cause of plateau. Bringing a higher-degree of relaxation into your core workout, brings a higher- degree of ability for your body to integrate its functional capacities. Relaxation is a critical functional capacity.

An expert marksman has integrated breath awareness to its subtleties. The more skilled he is with his core, the more skilled he is at breathing. The integral nature of relaxation, in the marksman's ability to achieve pin-point accuracy, requires possessing a functional ability to relax into the shot.

Body Integration

In terms of the One Minute Workout, as you are focusing into the contraction of the core, you are focusing relaxation into the rest of the body. Using only the appropriate level of strength to maintain a balanced posture throughout the entirety of the rest of the body where contraction is not the focus.

Section 4: Stretching

Maybe even more important than contraction and relaxation is stretching. In fact, if you are just getting back into exercise, focusing only on stretching may be the place to start. Specifically, the hips and thorax.

Stretching can combine both contraction and relaxation into one output of energy. As a muscle stretches, it must relax. As the muscle reaches it maximum elasticity, it begins to act with force to bring the muscle back into its "normal" range of movement. More than that, stretching appropriately can induce the tears in a muscle similar to how contraction does. This can be accomplished by an eccentric muscle contraction, where the motion of an active (contracting) muscle is lengthened due to load.

When done properly, stretching is the least invasive way to get fit. This theory of integrating the body considers stretching as massaging the body from the inside out. It activates muscles in such a way that is not possible through another form of activation.

In the same way that you use minor movements to find deeper contractions, you also use minor movements to find a deeper stretch. And in terms of tenseness and soreness in a muscle, stretching appropriately can bring relief to that area. And in severe cases of extended pain, when a muscle group begins to go numb due to over stimulation of pain, stretching is a guaranteed way to not only bring the life vitality of sensation back into the area, but also bring relief to the pain.

A significant majority of any muscle stretched will necessarily have corollaries in the core. The One Minute Workout takes advantage of this fact. In every movement you make throughout the day, you are engaging you core to some degree. Likewise, there is never a moment where you cannot find a way to stretch your core. It's possible to stretch your abdominals, back extensors, and obliques by taking a deep breath in. Likewise, it's possible to contract them all by squeezing the air from your lungs through contraction. This is the most basic form of the One Minute Workout. As you experiment with this workout, spend a day exploring all the way you can stretch your core, inside of what you already do. What are the micro movements you need to stretch your core at your desk, driving in your car, doing dishes, standing in line. And use your breath as the flashlight of discovery as you explore the dark jungle of unknown micromovements.

Section 5: Recovery

Intensity walks hand-in-hand with gentleness. There are very few systems that are designed to produce output at increased levels for extended periods. Intervals of maintenance and support are as justified as the intervals of intensity.

In many ways, stretching is both an exercise routine, and a recovery routine. In terms of the One Minute Workout, recovery is rather quick for these muscle groups. The muscles used in the One Minute Workout are postural muscles; meaning, they are always active, unless you're at a complete resting state where the muscles don't have to work to maintain your posture.

Before you go to sleep, take a moment to breathe deeply into these muscles and think, "let go". Generate gratitude reflecting on the stability they provide you to move through your day and create your life. Rest now, tomorrow you rise.

Body Integration

Section 6: Integration

Forward from this moment, all integration rests upon your root – the perineal-coccyx basis. The transfer of balance that occurs between the perineum and coccyx, is the first and most important transition of conscious awareness to refine. As a foundation to a house, the stability of your body transfers all movement through this point.

The first step to integration, is increasing sensate awareness off this transfer of physical energy from the root (perineum), through the tip of the tailbone (coccyx complex), and into the rest of the body. You can do this now. There is no excuse to not focus here and now except your decision not to. This degree of clarity is within your full control in every moment you become aware of your breath. You can bring awareness to this transfer point at any given time, during any activity. It is only your rationalization to *not* do it that has you not do it. Set aside the mental narratives you perpetuate. The decision is yours. Choose to do, or not do, and leave it at that.

Take a breath, and continue to breathe awareness through this transition point of the perineum and tip of the tailbone. Squeeze the perineum gently as you breathe in, and notice the physical sensation of energetic movement up the body. If you have trouble feeling this, intend to contract the gluteus muscles, and the back extensors. Contract only to the point needed to begin to feel physical sensation in this area, and hold the contraction.

Now release the contraction. Continue to sense. Hold sensate focus in this area. If you continue to struggle with being able to sense this area, begin a movement of flexion counter to the movement you just contracted. All you may need to do is move your chin towards your chest. Start with a small movement. Refine your sensate focus to the micro movements of your body. Dramatic shifts in angular orientation of your joints stimulates a

Body Integration

significant neurological activity, and thus, is easier to sense. Tip your head forward a centimeter and notice for any transfer of energy between your perineum and tailbone. Being to refine your sense-ability to this degree. You are increasing your sensitivity by doing this. **Be warned**, your emotions will become stronger as you move through this refinement. You must allow yourself the space to feel the fullness of your emotions in your own body. Until you make this decision, your emotional experience will always be subdued by the fear of feeling them fully.

Until you are at point where you have refined your sensation such that you can sense these micro movements throughout your core, there is potential to increase both your motor skills, as well as you emotional skills. If you have room to increase your motor skills, you can become a more skilled athlete. If you have room to increase your emotional skills, you can become a more skilled human.

The premise on which Body Integration rests, is that the living body is an athletic instrument that has the capacity for locomotion. The fuel for that locomotion is emotion. The emotion used can be passion, determination, joy, love, hate, anger, curiosity, or a combination of various emotional vectors. As such, every human is an athlete and has a capacity for refinement of both awareness of the body and the induction of motion. Inducing motion happens by way of generating emotion – motivation. You are encouraged to use joy as the motivator. Begin to orient your paradigm to a *joy of movement*.

The pursuit of your happiness is within your full control. Your breath will show you the way.

Body Integration | Phase 2: Learning to Love the Body You're In

"The journey toward sustainable joy happens in the vehicle of my body..."

Section 1: Emotional Resilience

As it pertains to being human, harnessing the power of emotions is both a skill set to be mastered, as well as a state-of-being that allows for increased quality of experience. The converse, emotional stagnancy, is the root of suffering in the human experience. When emotional energy is not allowed to fully process, the resulting blockage in the body presents itself as physical tension of some sort. Whether the tension is a knotted muscle, or a hardened artery, emotional blockage exists due to lifestyle choices. These choices are results of an individual's paradigm in life. Orienting to a new paradigm is a goal of *body integration*. In this way, "body integration" can be defined as the synergy of the mental, emotional, and physical bodies through the vehicle of awareness.

Placing distinct attention into the shoulders and hips is a first step of orienting to body integration. For the shoulders, this includes the ribs, the shoulder blades, the humerus bone, the cervical vertebrae, and all connecting tissues, muscles, fascia, tendons, etc. For the hips this includes the femur, the pelvic bone, the hip blades, the vertebrae of the lumbar, and all connecting tissues, muscles, fascia, tendons, etc.

All these periphery elements are included as part of the shoulders and hips precisely because these elements are either directly linked to the areas, as is the case the cervical and lumbar areas; or the elements compose these regions, as is the case with the shoulder and hip blades. In short, any part of your body that is itself part of the shoulder or hip or is directly connected to the shoulder or hip by muscle, fascia, etc. is involved with integrating these areas of the body. And if you notice your movement, these two areas, the shoulders and hips, significantly influence movement of every other part of your body. Housed between the shoulders and the hips are all your vital organs except the brain. The *most important* element for *integration* that is housed between these two – the diaphragm[1].

Section 2: Facing the Pain

Residual pain acts as signal. A point of focus in the practice of body integration. An unavoidable signal. Except when the residual pain is chronic such that the senses begin to numb.

Focusing into these pain-points acts as a movement toward identifying root-causes. Doctors who advise symptom relief *without* addressing the underlying cause are of a certain medical practice. Doctors who advise addressing the underlying cause, are of another type of medical practice. Identifying the root of issues in life requires going beyond being only aware of symptoms. Symptomatic relief is **not** a goal of *body integration* though it is a benefit, nonetheless.

As a point of note, the distinction of pain as result of improper movement and posture while engaging a practice is something to avoid. The difference between **residual pain** as way of lifestyle choices, genetic disposition, or some form of trauma induced on the body, and **pain** that results from not moving in symmetry with a joint's functional range are two different aspects of human experience.

---

[1] https://www.ncbi.nlm.nih.gov/pmc/articles/PMC3731110/

Body Integration

Understanding the difference in addressing each of these types of pain signals is a significant aspect of integrating the wisdom of the body. In the case of residual pain, its finally listening to what the body has been telling you. In the case of immediate pain induced by improper movement, it's an opportunity to take a step back from the idea you're moving with to re-assess your approach toward more gentleness and ease. In the context of "facing the pain", this is a movement to begin unwinding habituated ignorance of your body's somatic experience. The degree to which you resist the idea that you've been ignorant is the degree to which you resist your own body's wisdom. Succumbing to pride in this resistance is counterproductive to the overall goal of increasing your quality of life. Open yourself to move with dignified humility.

2.1 Inflammation

In flame is inflammation. And it is the body's way to deal with unwanted invaders, burn them out. However, when the body goes into over drive, and turns into a pyro-maniac, inflammation becomes the enemy. Particularly, inflammation of the fascia of the body[2].

If you've ever dissected mammalian muscle tissue, you know that fascia is wrapped around everything. It is the connective tissue that keeps the body from falling into a lumpy liquid pile. Additionally, fascia has nerve endings. **Lots and lots of nerve endings**[3]. Imagine if the fascia becomes inflamed beyond what is normal?

---

[2] https://www.doctorschierling.com/blog/more-on-the-inflammation-fibrosis-scar-tissue-connection
[3] https://www.doctorschierling.com/blog/why-fascia-twenty-reasons-why-fascia

2.2 Relaxed Shoulders and Hips

Tight shoulders and hips act as a signal for undiscovered residual pain. Prolonged muscular rigidity in these areas acts to mold the body into a certain shape. The joints get pulled in certain directions. The bones tilt at specific angles. And as the body becomes cast to this posture, it is stretching and moving the body in dynamic ways, toward opening into a more fluid range of joint movement, that enhances one's freedom. In this case, its freedom of movement.

Whether its stretching, myofascial release, slow discrete movement with the breath, or some form of muscular exercise; tuning into the shoulders, hips, and the spine that connects the two, as a focus toward reducing pain and increasing suppleness begins to reshape the dominant body-mold. How the body is held throughout the day, especially in moments of unconsciousness of the body, is a primary source of prolonged discomfort if the body-posture is not conducive toward a sense of ease[4].

Stabilizing the body into a posture-of-ease as the pre-dominant body-base is a distinct goal of body integration. *Sensing* into this posture of ease **requires** facing the pain in the hip and shoulder joints such that the joints and bones in these areas are allowed to move into a basis of ease.

2.3 Stabilized Feet

Autonomous locomotion of the body, independent of external aid, is best facilitated through the feet. There may be some who can walk on their hands, and some yet who have no other option but to use something other than the feet. As a design, the human body is intended to use the feet to move with the highest degree of speed, agility, power, and many other force appliers, such as

---

[4] https://www.nutritiousmovement.com/a-list-of-body-casts/

Body Integration

grace. Locomotion of the human body is made possible by the feet.

As such, proper attention must be given to this most useful tool. As the stresses and tensions of life drain themselves to the feet, the entirety of the body's posture is necessarily impacted. Proper posture of the body is **highly influence** through proper posture of the feet, even when sitting and laying. In many types of movement, where the feet go, the hips follow. And in other type of movements, the reverse is also true, where the hips go, the feet follow. Studying this synergy as a sensate-focus begins to process a most critical function of body integration – grounding.

As an energetic system, the body needs a way to drain off excess energy, fluctuations in intensities, and disturbances in frequencies. The feet act as that drain, or grounding rod. Imagine a shower drain full of hair. The energy still drains, but at a significantly reduced capacity. If a severe clog is present, the water stands stagnant in the tub. The same is true of the many different types of energies moving through the body.

One of those is emotional energy. Specifically, the emotion of stress. In this context, "stress" is a broad categorization of the emotional energies that induce a state of dis-ease in the body; depression, resentments, fears, frustrations, anger, rage, grief, guilt, shame, jealousy, self-loathing, anxiety, etc.

The situational context acting as a trigger for the emotional resonance can be, and is often, a multi-factor variable. "Standing firm" in the emotional resilience to feel the fullness of the situation is facilitated by an integrated exploration of the feet. Reflexology is a known method to begin that exploration.

In this context, "reflexology" is nothing more than studying the manipulation of the points in the foot that allows for a release of tension. This may come through a self-administered foot massage, or a pair of in-soles that facilitate a proper bone

Body Integration

alignment of the feet. The mechanism used to integrate the foot is less important than the act of exploring the *sense* of integration.

2.4 Supple Jaw

Relaxed jaw, as opposed to grinding teeth. Fluid movement as opposed to tight contractions. These variances typify what it means to have a *supple* jaw. The subtle nuance where attention need be focus is what's the state of the jaw when you're not aware of it. This paradox is similar to the wave-particle duality of light. Is it a particle or a wave? It seems to depend on your observation. When you become aware of the state of your jaw, it can change the state of your jaw. The key is to take note of the state at the initial moment of cognizance. If its tight, and the teeth are clenched, take note of anything in the environment that may be acting as an influence on how you are holding your jaw. If there is nothing that is necessarily influencing the state of your jaw, it can be said that this is the average state of your jaw. If its tight, constricted, and rigid, there's work to be done on moving toward suppleness.

A factor to include in contemplation of your movement toward integrating your jaw is informed by an assessment of how the residual stress of a tight jaw acts as a force contrary to proper alignment of your body. How does clenching the teeth influence the atlas at the top of the spine? How does tight jaw muscles influence the muscles of the neck? What are the correlations of a tight jaw to any pain/discomforts in the neck? How does pain in the neck influence the posture of the rest of your spine? And how does the posture of your spine influence the rest of your body? Exploring these correlations through the process by which you integrate your body *is* your practice of body-integration.

2.5 Sensitive Hands

Sensing the subtle sensations of the body is a skill to be developed. The pads of the fingertips act as point of focus in

Body Integration

refinement of this skill. Increasing the sensitivity of the perceptive mechanism allows for a more acute identification of the pain points in the body. Join the tip of the pad of each finger to the thumb with a full breath cycle, both inhale and exhale. Sensing the subtleties of this focus facilitates a sharpening of the mind.

Managing the attention point toward noticing the subtle sensations, and variation of sensation, both during the breath-cycle on a particular finger, as well as the variation from one finger to the next, is the process of refinement. As your ability to notice these variations increase, so too does your capacity to notice a variation of sensation throughout the rest of your body. This skill is critical as it pertains to being microscopic in your movements as you assess the current state of you body-integrity, as well as move into a more robust integration.

As the sensitivity of your fingertips increase, so to does the overall sensitivity of your hands. As the overall sensitivity of your hands increase, so to does the overall sensitivity of the rest of your body. Being sensitive to the subtle nuance of environments and situations is the basis of what it means to be emotionally intelligent. Being emotionally intelligent in situations acts a basis for both resolving conflict, as well as increasing collaboration and synergy.

Section 3: Breath Integrity
Breath is the single most important function the body uses to survive. The body can last weeks without food, days without water, hours as the blood drains; but if the capacity to breath is taken away, the body dies in minutes. Furthermore, of all the involuntary body processes to sustain your life, breath is the only one that you can both directly control, and also be unconscious of control while it functions sufficiently.

Body Integration

Experimentation of the theory espoused in this book has the pre-requisite of being able to focus the locus of air intake at the bottom of the larynx, near the top of the trachea. Breathing with a focus of air intake centered anywhere else above the larynx does not allow for being at the root of the systems input mechanism. That's not to say that breathing from another area should not be done. This pre-requisite is saying that developing the conscious ability to bring air in, by controlling the flow at its base is a necessary skill to see the fullness of body integration come to life. To gain full unbiased observation in your experimentation/practice, breathing in this way is necessary. Breathing in others ways will be useful in your practice, but this "base breath" will be used as the main mechanism to bring the mind's focus into the body's sensations.

Imagine slowly breathing in the fragrance of a flower. Keep the mouth closed and allow the air to move into your nose ever so delicately. When done properly, you will hear and ocean-wind sound coming from your throat. If you suck in through the nose, you will hear the sound the from nose.

Close the mouth, open the air passageways, and contract the diaphragm. Air will be pulled into the lungs as a vacuum pressure. The diaphragm pulls the lungs down and open creating the vacuum pressure. In the vacuum is where choice is fostered by way of intent-full awareness.

3.1 Guiding the Breath

Being unconscious of breathing is also called autonomic-breathing. And as defined herein this theory, being conscious of breathing is referred to as an infusion. As oxygen is infused into the lungs, the diaphragm acts as the force-applier of the breathing function. Allowing an infusion of air into the lungs is facilitating the tensor-equilibrium in the diaphragm. As a tensor function, the diaphragm can be allowed to both tighten around the internal structures, as well as stretch those same structures.

Generally speaking, most humans, as they yawn, experience an increase of upward force on the bottom of the rib cage as the internal air pressure is drawn through the breath into the lower lungs. The yawning function can simultaneously contract the diaphragm, stretch the abdominals, and contract the intercostals muscles of the upper rib cage. This type of function in the diaphragm is a typical scenario.

Diaphragmatic attenuation, however, is a process whereby the diaphragm is stretched through proprioceptive neuromuscular facilitation (PNF). This method draws air into the full functional capacity of the lungs wherein the diaphragm contracts but is also forced to stretch through subtle movements. Refining the ability to effectively use the diaphragm is critical to releasing tension bound in the muscles, fascia, tendons, and ligaments throughout the entirety of the body. Diaphragmatic attenuation is both a reduction of the manifest tension in the diaphragm, as well as a strengthening of it.

The process of ingesting air into the stomach in a passive manner, by way of increasing the elasticity of the diaphragm is a sign that tension is being released. The diaphragm will not relax if there is tension being held in the body. As tension is released, it becomes possible to passively ingest air. This helps to expand the internal organs, creating an internal pressure that facilitates a body posture toward a net positive posture. Increasing relaxation by decreasing the strain on various joints by way of diaphragmatic relaxation can happen through a deep proprioceptive awareness of those internal systems. This is a method to slow the breath, without *forcing* the breath to slow down. This type of *breath awareness* is an effective method of "allowing the breath to guide you".

Body Integration

Integrity of the breathing function can be developed by following 4 primary movements to induce integration of the breath. Those movements for this protocol of *breath induction* are 1) Deep, 2) Full, 3) Slow, and 4) Long.

1. Deep: consciously breathing into the lower section of the lungs such that the movement results in the expansion of the belly.
2. Full: focusing the movement of the inhale toward the functional max intake of air into the lungs.
3. Slow: breathing at a pace that is 10 times the pace of a regular autonomic breath.
4. Long: allowing the posture of the front of the body to open *with* the inhale, such that the jaw drops, the rib cage lifts, and the abdominals lengthen.

As these four breath-movements integrate into a symmetry of motion, *and* as the mind is allowed to focus into specific points of the body that require a release of tension, it can be said that one's breathing has reached a point of integrity. The more these breath movements merge into one singular focus, the more the mind is allowed to focus on the periphery movements of the body (legs, arms, neck, back, etc.) in greater degrees of awareness. Using these 4 breath-functions to explore the movements of the rest of body is a way to call forth a self-awareness otherwise impossible. As self-awareness of the blockages in the body become clear, so too does the opportunity to find full resolution of those stagnancies of energy that have been held in the body.

If performing this breath, a yawn is triggered, allow the yawn to happen. The Breath Induction Protocol mechanically facilitates yawning. The purpose of this protocol is to use the fullness of your lungs while in a proprioceptive awareness of your body's movement. *Allow the yawn to happen.* Yawning is process by which your body releases tension. Focus on the majority of the

Body Integration

inhale to be through the nose as described above. If yawning is induced, take in as much through the nose as is possible, then allow the jaw to open such that the yawn can take full effect. Inhale the remainder through the mouth. Exhale by pursing the lips to a small aperture and breathe out as is comfortable in the due course of the yawn.

Both guide the breath and let the breath guide you. Be both a leader and a follower. Discern the nuance of trusting your body herein the movement of breathing.

3.2 Breathing Open the Shoulders and Hips

Using the base-breath as described above, both with the locus of control at the bottom of the larynx, and using the four movements of breath awareness, inhale and notice the sensations in the shoulders. Relax into the exhale. And move into another inhale, this time focusing on the hips.

Allow the sensations in these two areas to come into the spotlight of your awareness. Notice for any sensations that you've been disregarding or setting aside. Allow these sensations to be felt. Visualize your breath as cool water flowing through these areas.

Continue with this breathing for 5 more breaths. Alternating each inhale between the hips and the shoulders. **If you feel a need to stand and rotate the hips**, follow the guidance of your body. **If you feel a need to raise your arms up around in the air to open the chest**, follow the guidance of your body. If you feel the posture and movement you are currently in could be repositioned or manipulated in some way to facilitate more ease in your breathing, follow the guidance of your body.

There is no specific routine defined here other than using your breath to tune into the nuances of your body. In doing so, you allow your body to tell you what it needs. This is much more different that being in your head trying to figure out what position

Body Integration

you should put your body in to practice a yoga pose, or a tai chi movement, or some exercise routine. Your body knows what it needs. You must simply give it the opportunity to speak to you in a way that you are able to hear it and heed its guidance.

3.3 Breathing Into the Feet

Using the base-breath as described above, both with the locus of control at the bottom of the larynx, and using the four movements of breath awareness, inhale and notice the sensations in the feet. Relax into the exhale. And move into another inhale.

Allow the sensations in the feet to come into the spotlight of your awareness. Notice for any sensations that you've been disregarding or setting aside. Allow these sensations to be felt. Visualize your breath as cool water flowing through these areas.

Continue with this breathing for 5 more breaths. Alternating each inhale between the hips, the shoulders and feet. **If you feel a need to stand and spread your toes by the weight of your body**, follow the guidance of your body. **If you feel a need to sit and massage the pressure points of your feet**, follow the guidance of your body. If you feel the posture and movement you are currently in could be repositioned or manipulated in some way to facilitate more ease in your breathing, follow the guidance of your body.

There is no specific routine defined here other than using your breath to tune into the nuances of your body. In doing so, you allow your body to tell you what it needs. This is much more different than being in your head trying to figure out what position you should put your body in to practice a yoga pose, or a tai chi movement, or some exercise routine. Your body knows what it needs. You must simply give it the opportunity to speak to you in a way that you are able to hear it and heed its guidance.

Body Integration

3.4 Breathing Down the Jaw

Using the base-breath as described above, both with the locus of control at the bottom of the larynx, and using the four movements of breath awareness, inhale and notice the sensations in the jaw. Relax into the exhale. And move into another inhale.

Allow the sensations in the jaw to come into the spotlight of your awareness. Notice for any sensations that you've been disregarding or setting aside. Allow these sensations to be felt. Visualize your breath as cool water flowing through these areas.

Continue with this breathing for 5 more breaths. Alternating each inhale between the hips, the shoulders, the feet, and the jaw. **If you feel a need to open your mouth and drop your jaw as if you were yawning**, follow the guidance of your body. **If you feel a need to gently tap with your fingers on your jaw and jaw bones**, follow the guidance of your body. If you feel the posture and movement you are currently in could be repositioned or manipulated in some way to facilitate more ease in your breathing, follow the guidance of your body.

There is no specific routine defined here other than using your breath to tune into the nuances of your body. In doing so, you allow your body to tell you what it needs. This is much more different than being in your head trying to figure out what position you should put your body in to practice a yoga pose, or a tai chi movement, or some exercise routine. Your body knows what it needs. You must simply give it the opportunity to speak to you in a way that you are able to hear it and heed its guidance.

3.5 Breathing Through the Palms

Using the base-breath as described above, both with the locus of control at the bottom of the larynx, and using the four movements of breath awareness, inhale and notice the sensations in the hands. Relax into the exhale. And move into another inhale.

Body Integration

Allow the sensations in the hands to come into the spotlight of your awareness. Notice for any sensations that you've been disregarding or setting aside. Allow these sensations to be felt. Visualize your breath as cool water flowing through these areas.

Continue with this breathing for 10 more breaths. Alternating each inhale between the hips, the shoulders, the feet, the jaw, and the hands. **If you feel a need to spread your fingers wide while rotating your wrists,** follow the guidance of your body. **If you feel a need to massage the muscle between the index and thumb**, follow the guidance of your body. If you feel the posture and movement you are currently in could be repositioned or manipulated in some way to facilitate more ease in your breathing, follow the guidance of your body.

There is no specific routine defined here other than using your breath to tune into the nuances of your body. In doing so, you allow your body to tell you what it needs. This is much more different than being in your head trying to figure out what position you should put your body in to practice a yoga pose, or a tai chi movement, or some exercise routine. Your body knows what it needs. You must simply give it the opportunity to speak to you in a way that you are able to hear it and heed its guidance.

Section 4: Posture Equilibrium

Posture is neither static nor rigid.

Contemplate that for a moment.

Take a moment right now and explore the 4 movements of *breath induction* discussed previously. Full, deep, long, slow. Breathe while contemplating that **posture is neither static nor rigid.**

After you have completed one cycle of breath induction with the previous contemplation, take another cycle of breath induction while contemplating the notion of *equilibrium* as a somatic

Body Integration

experience in your joints. Notice if you sense a desire to shift the body toward equilibrium as you contemplate this. Be aware if it's the suggestion to notice that induced the desire, or if the desire is resonant regardless of the suggestion.

Analysis of the posture happens through inspecting the dynamics of one's joint stability, flexibility, and range of movement. In the analysis, there will painful sensations, pleasurable sensations, and a host of other various sensations. Navigating through these sensations is the journey of learning to love the body you're in. The release of tension is a very specific type of sensation to be able to sense toward while performing the analysis. The result of such analysis is the development of an active process to lessen the degree of rigidity that persists in the shoulders, hips, jaw, hands, and feet, etc; and increase latent fluidity and suppleness thereof.

When performing the initial breath above, while contemplating that posture is neither rigid nor static, you may have noticed the axiomatic nature of your breath. Proper posture for *breathing*, **cannot** be static or rigid. The breath is in constant motion. Unless it's being consciously held in the lungs; in which case, breathing has consequently stopped. As such, the **posture** of breathing *is itself* a **movement**.

Breathing does not happen without moving.

Structural analysis and manipulation toward proper bone alignment is fundamentally tied to breathing. As the lungs fill and empty of air, the ribs move. As the ribs move, so do the costovertebral joints; that which connects the rib to the spine. The result of which is that when breath happens, the spine moves. As the spine moves, so too does the rest of body. The interdependency here is self-evident.

The ribs protect the lungs and heart. The lungs clean the blood so the brain can stay active. As the brain stays active it helps to

Body Integration

regulate the pumping of the heart. As the heart pumps the body maintains life vitality.

As such, posture is a ***process.***

One such process to move with is *equilibrium*. There are many different types of processes that one can move with. It's a matter of choosing one and implementing it. In-deed the body is currently processing a type of posture as it reads this. All that's needed is a decision to *allow* it the opportunity to *sense* toward equilibrium.

The experimentations described below act as opportunities to explore each area of the body in a movement toward equilibrium. **As a sensation in the body.**

4.1 Posture of the Hips

Stand, positioning the feet, slightly wider than the hips, knees with a slight bend. The tip of each toe touching the ground. The pad and the heel of each foot carrying a balanced load of weight.

Imagine a string connected to the perineum, drawn straight to the ground between your feet. Now imagine a small coin lying in the center between the feet, directly below the end of the string. Begin rotating your hips in either direction, ever so slightly such that the very end of the string circles the coin. Move through **3** breath induction cycles while rotating, then pause, and begin to slowly rotate the hips in the other direction for **3** breaths. Still keeping the end of the string circling that circumference of the coin.

After 3 breaths circling the coin in both directions, imagine a donut where the coin was and repeat the process. Rotate the hips with **3** full, slow, long, deep breaths in each direction, so the imaginary string circles the imaginary donut.

Body Integration

Now imagine a frisbee, and repeat the triad of breath cycles, circling the frisbee.

And now a basketball. Breathe. Rotate.

All the while sensing for proper posture of **Your** hips.

Now begin to decrease the circumference, slowly spiraling back to the size of a small coin in whichever direction you find yourself rotating.

If you yawn, you're doing it correctly. You may find yourself yawning frequently, this is ok. Allow the breath to breath.

4.2 Posture of the Shoulders

Stand or sit with the spine upright, the chin high such that the bottom of the jawbone is parallel with ground. Chest raised with the arms hanging gently at the sides.

Begin a breath induction cycle and gently rotate the inside of both elbows to the front, keeping the arm generally straight at the side. If the arm is completely straight so the crease of the elbow is flat, increase the gentleness by releasing the contraction in the triceps. Find the point that elbow won't rotate further without pain. Now, rotate gently in the opposite direction such that the elbow hanging at the side rotates to the back. Again, find the point it won't rotate any further without contracting the triceps. Do not forcefully exert the rotation to the point of pain in the joint. Microscopically move with the subtle nuance of gentleness.

Continue breathing deep, long, slow, and full while slowly rotating forward and backward. Now being slowly raising the arms to the sides while continuing to alternate the rotation.

Breath. Alternate rotation. And raise the arms until they are straight overhead, or you have found that maximum point at which your shoulders will raise. If they don't go all the way

Body Integration

overhead, that is okay, **do not** force it. This is a process of gently exploring the subtlety of your shoulder socket.

Continue breathing while alternating rotation, and slowly lower your arms to back down to gently hand at your side.

Again, if you yawn, you're doing it correctly. Pause if you need to such that you can more effectively let the yawn be as full as it needs to be. Remember, yawning is process by which your body releases tension. In this case, it is the tension of your shoulders.

When in doubt, yawn it out.

4.3 Posture of the Feet

Sit with the spine upright, the legs in a 90-degree angle at the knee, with the feet slightly wider that shoulder width. Place the heel on the ground and raise the front of the foot off the ground while keeping your toes extended straight out.

Begin a breath induction cycle, while slowly lowering the inside of each foot so the joint of the big toe that connects it to the foot gently touches the ground. Continue breathing while slowly and softly lowering the big toe so the tip gently rests on the ground. Now lower the next toe so only the tip touches the ground. Continue lowering each toe in like manner while breathing. Focus on moving only one toe at a time resting each on the ground. If you notice difficulty in moving only one toe, this is ok, its an indication that you require more practice of proprioception in this way.

As the pinky toe touches the ground, allow the big toe to slowly raise. Followed in succession by each toe until only the side of your foot is resting on the ground.

Again, if you're unable to rotate the ankle in such a way, **do not** force it. Simply move to the ankle's rotational maximum. Also note that one ankle may be able to rotate more than the other.

Body Integration

This is ok. There is no predefined maximum that you should target as your goal. The **goal** as such is to give yourself the opportunity to explore the subtlety of your ankle while breathing deeply in this somatic journey of self-awareness. As you practice, you will notice that your joint's maximum may find a wider range of movement. Or you may already be at your functional maximum, and find that as you practice this, you discover a more integrated flow of bio-electrical sensation in your feet. There is no predefined thing that you will discover. Discovery as such is unique to each individual.

With the blade of your foot's edge resting on the ground, begin another breath and slowly rotate the ankle back inward such that pink toe touches first, followed successively by each toe thereafter. Rotate inward to the big toe and allow the pinky toe to raise off the ground until only the big to is touching. Now raise the front of the foot up back to the starting position with toes extend out straight. Spread them as wide as is comfortable. Repeat this for at least two more rotation cycles.

When in doubt, yawn it out.

4.4 Posture of the Hands

While inhaling, open the hands as wide as you possibly can. Fully extend the fingers. Now exhale and relax the fingers to move back into a comfortable open position such that no part of any finger is touching.

Begin a breath induction cycle, inhaling while bringing the index finger and thumb together such that the tips of each gently touch. Move the fingers in synchronicity with the breath in such a way that the breath reaches the max inhale as the fingers begin to touch. Let the fingers rest for a moment as you begin the exhale slowly returning both the index and the thumb to its original relaxed position.

Body Integration

Inhale again while slowly moving the middle finger and thumb together in similar manner to as before. Bring them together just as the inhale reaches its max. Pause. And slowly exhale returning each to its original position.

Continue in this fashion for each finger.

As you finish with the exhale on the pinky, begin another breath, bringing the index, middle, and ring fingers together to touch the thumb in similar manner as above. The connection happens as the breath reaches its max. Leave the pinky comfortably extended such that it does not touch any other finger. Now exhale and return the fingers to their original position.

As you practice, notice for where you hold tension in the movement. Relax the wrist and forearms and move into a sense of release of the tension as the fingers move together, slowly curling together to touch as the breath reaches its max.

If you notice difficulty synchronizing the movement of the fingers and the breath, this is ok. It's an indicator that a greater degree of self-awareness is available. By practicing this you're doing exactly what you need to in order to develop that awareness.

4.5 Posture of the Jaw

Before beginning this exercise, it is recommended that you practice both the Breath Induction Protocol to a proficiency, as well as the above exercise for posture. A significant degree of tension can be held in the jaw. It's advisable to ensure the rest of the body has processed toward an openness such that tension in the jaw can more effectively release. Holding tension in other parts of the body, in a certain sense, is holding tension in the jaw. For example, when experiencing sharp pain anywhere in the body, and a quick inhale is triggered, notice what the jaw does.

For this exercise, while doing the breath induction protocol, rather than inhaling through the nose, inhale through the mouth.

Body Integration

Still with the locus of control at the bottom of the larynx, near the top of the trachea. Slowly open the mouth by extending the bottom jawbone down and out in a gentle, slow, movement.

Yawning in this exercise is the goal.

Open the belly and the let air come in while contracting the coccygeus to a subtle 10% contraction.

Continue breathing in this way while endeavoring to have each successive breath be a yawn. Develop the ability to breathe ten consecutive yawns.

If it feels more comfortable to begin the inhale through the nose, this is ok. When the lungs are approximately one-third full, begin to move to breathe the remainder of the breath through the mouth.

If nearing the top of the inhale, and you sense a subdued yawn, where it feels like you can breathe deeper but are unable, slow the intake of air, and relax the jaw open and further down. If that doesn't allow the yawn to take full effect, continue breathing in as **deeply as you possibly can**. And exhale allowing your body to relax, letting the exhale take care of itself. If this subdued sense persists, it's an indicator that there is tension held somewhere else in the body and more exploration of your body's tensions is needed.

If, after exhaling, you feel a need to swallow, do so.

If, after exhaling, you feel a need to suck in quickly through your nose, do so. But do not exhale thereafter. Move into slowly inhaling in the manner of a breath induction.

If, while executing ten consecutive breaths, you find yourself distracted, or justifying a reason to not do ten breaths, be cognizant of irrational excuses justifying the cessation of the exploration. Discerning the difference between an irrational

Body Integration

excuse and a valid justification is the nuanced journey of learning to love the body you're in. Succumb not to irrational excuse. *Move in the integrity of humbling yourself to the dignity of wisdom inherent to honoring your body's needs.*

Most importantly, while breathing these ten yawns, be sure to put awareness in the jaw such that you notice where there is tension, where there is relaxation, where there is pleasure, where there is pain. Notice the nuance of as many sensations as possible. Also notice other areas of the body where sensation is triggered as you yawn. This somatic awareness acts as a sensate visibility to the interdependent relationship of systems composing the body.

Section 5: Tension Analysis and Release

In many ways, residual tension is a result of unprocessed stress. Inasmuch as the tension is residual, is as much as the tension is based on a habit of not processing stress in the body. In this context, the term "stress" is broadly defined as anything that inhibits an ease of life experience. It could be physical stress, emotional stress, mental stress, or any combination thereof. The habit could be as simple as sitting for prolonged periods in a bone-alignment that puts undue stress on the lower back. The degree of unconsciousness habituated in the movements and postures is the degree to which tension has a place to reside in the body over the long term.

Making a deliberate choice to place attention on the somatic nuance of tension, and more importantly, its release, acts as a pattern interrupt to the habituated program running in consciousness. **Decisions** as such are the sole responsibility of the one inhabiting the body. In-habiting implies an intrinsic patterning process. If you are inhabiting a body, you are sole possessor of the decisioning process. This process of making choice is a constancy. Choices are always being made.

Body Integration

To reiterate the point of this section: the degree of unconsciousness habituated in the movements and postures is the degree to which tension has a place to reside in the body over the long term. Repatterning of unconsciousness happens through a trajectory of choices **yet to be made**. Awareness of the choice is a pre-condition to making the choice. What reminders are in place in your environment that act as influences toward this repatterning?

Analysis of the pockets of tension is best facilitated by the breath. Breathing into these areas begins to shine the light of awareness such that the tension can be released. The method expressed herein for such breathing is based on both the Core Focus sequence and the Breath Induction protocol. With these two practices as the basis, the final ingredient is facilitating a proprioceptive awareness of a neuromuscular release of tension.

The goal is to build the skill of tuning into the minutia of somatic equilibrium in such a way where you, as the facilitator of release, allow your body to mechanically override the tension. This is the "neuromuscular facilitation". Muscles act in specific predictable ways. Inducing muscular relaxation, by way of overriding the neurological reactive mechanism that keeps muscle in a state of rigidity, requires a commitment to being gentle with the body. As such, this is an opportunity to develop deep self-compassion. This method is not "forcing" the body to adapt to your wishes. This is not a "mind over matter" exertion of will power. This is using bio-mechanical processes to heighten your sensitivity of awareness wherein you facilitate the rise of relaxation.

It bears repeating, this method DOES NOT WORK through forcing yourself. It requires being gentle with yourself. In this you will come to face any long-harbored self-esteem issues you may have. Noticing the narratives that arise suggesting something counter to self-compassion, are the precise cognitive-emotional

Body Integration

configurations you are working to restore to a state of equilibrium. You can call this "shadow-work" if you like. Regardless, that which you have harbored, resting at the base of the unconscious cognitive-emotional configurations, presenting as somatic tension, pain, or general discomfort, are the precise body-points to breath into.

For the experimentations described below, the names of the muscles are given such that the terms can be easily referenced online. Research as needed to gain understanding of the precise location of each muscle.

5.1 Shoulder Analysis and Release

Sit or stand in a comfortable position. Begin by using the fingers of your hand to explore the top of the opposite side's Pectoralis Major just under the clavicle, for muscular tension, knots, or points where pain is unduly residing. All the while breathing in a slow, deep, full manner. In this case, breathing long is not necessary. The mechanical force applied by the fingers under the clavicle acts in similar manner to breathing long. Explore this area for at least 3 breaths.

If you find a point that is particularly tense or tightly knotted, pause on that point for a full breath, increasing the pressure to as much as is bearable but not excruciating.

Now switch hands and explore the other Pectoralis Major just under clavicle in similar manner as before.

Continue to breath, switching back to the other hand moving it up to the back, on the opposite side's Trapezius and begin exploring, with adequate pressure, feeling for knots in the muscle. Notice for the difference of tension in the trapezius and Rhomboid Minor. Explore this area for at least 3 breaths.

Now switch hands and move to explore the other trapezius and rhomboid minor as described above.

If a yawn is induced, allow it to be.

5.2 Hip Analysis and Release

Stand, sit, or lay in a comfortable position. Begin by using the fingers of each hand to explore its corresponding Gluteus Medius (left hand for the left hip, right for the right), for muscular tension, knots, or points where pain is unduly residing. All the while breathing in a slow, deep, full, and long manner. Explore this area for at least 3 breaths.

If you find a point that is particularly tense or tightly knotted, pause on that point for a full breath, increasing the pressure to as much as is bearable but not excruciating.

Now move into the Gluteus Maximus. You may need to shift positions to explore this area. Move to a comfortable position that allows you to use pressure to explore for muscular tension, etc. Explore this area for at least 3 breaths.

This may require you to explore only one side at a time.

Now move into exploring the Tensor Fasciae Latae. You may need to shift positions to explore this area. Move to a comfortable position that allows you to use pressure to explore for muscular tension, etc. Explore this area for at least 3 breaths.

Now move into exploring the Adductor Longus, as well as the Gracilis. You may need to shift positions to explore this area. Move to a comfortable position that allows you to use pressure to explore for muscular tension, etc. Explore this area for at least 3 breaths. **Note**, that if you begin to feel sexual sensations, this is ok. This exploration may induce those sensations; however, this is **not** an exercise of sexual exploration. Be discerning toward continuing to explore for muscular tension, knots, or points where pain is unduly residing.

If, while exploring, a yawn is induced, allow it to be.

Body Integration

5.3 Foot Analysis and Release

Sit in a comfortable position such that you can bring your foot into a position to hold it comfortably. Begin by using the fingers of either hand to explore the Adductor Hallucis, for muscular tension, knots, or points where pain is unduly residing. All the while breathing in a slow, deep, full, and long manner. Explore this area for at least 3 breaths.

If you find a point that is particularly tense or tightly knotted, pause on that point for a full breath, increasing the pressure to as much as is bearable but not excruciating.

Now move into exploring the Lumbrical muscles of the foot. You may need to shift positions to explore this area. Move to a comfortable position that allows you to use pressure to explore for muscular tension, etc. Explore this area for at least 3 breaths.

Now move into exploring the Quadratus Plantae and Adductor Digiti Minimi muscles of the foot. You may need to shift positions to explore this area. Move to a comfortable position that allows you to use pressure to explore for muscular tension, etc. Explore this area for at least 3 breaths.

If, while exploring, a yawn is induced, allow it to be.

5.4 Jaw Analysis and Release

Walk, stand, sit, or lay in a comfortable position. Begin by using the fingers of each hand to explore its corresponding Masseter Superficial (left hand for the left jaw, right for the right), for muscular tension, knots, or points where pain is unduly residing. All the while breathing in a slow, deep, full, and long manner. Explore this area for at least 3 breaths.

If you find a point that is particularly tense or tightly knotted, pause on that point for a full breath, increasing the pressure to as much as is bearable but not excruciating.

Body Integration

Now move into exploring the Risorius, and Depressor Anguli Oris muscles of the jaw. Explore this area for at least 3 breaths.

Now move into exploring the Platysma as it attaches to the bottom of the Mandible. Explore this area for at least 3 breaths.

If, while exploring, a yawn is induced, allow it to be.

5.5 Hand Analysis and Release

Walk, stand, sit, or lay in a comfortable position. Begin by using the fingers of one hand to explore the Dorsal Interossei and Adductor Pollicis of the other hand, for muscular tension, knots, or points where pain is unduly residing. All the while breathing in a slow, deep, full, and long manner. Explore this area for at least 3 breaths.

If you find a point that is particularly tense or tightly knotted, pause on that point for a full breath, increasing the pressure to as much as is bearable but not excruciating.

Now move into exploring the Opponens Pollicis, and Flexor Pollicis Brevis muscles of the hand. Explore this area for at least 3 breaths.

Now move into exploring the Abductor Digit Minimi and Flexor Digiti Minimi Brevis of the hand. Explore this area for at least 3 breaths.

If, while exploring, a yawn is induced, allow it to be.

Switch hands and begin exploring the other hand as described above.

Section 6: Emotional Integrity

The root of emotional integrity lies in the ability to have an emotional experience in the time frame the emotion arises, process the emotion, be able to respond to the situation with wisdom, and make decisions as necessary *without* removing

Body Integration

yourself. A less refined variation of that integrity is similar but rather than remaining in the situation to process, you remove yourself from the situation using effective and constructive communication such that other parties in the situation are given an awareness of the fact you need space and time to process. This less refined variation is still honoring yourself, however, the integration of your emotional body has yet to reach a state such that there is a simultaneous synergy of your ability to respond effectively in a given situation.

Using honesty in every situation means that, even if you have for yourself the goal of emotional integrity as described above, you sense the thresholds of your emotional capacities reached such that you feel a need to remove yourself from a situation; making the necessary accommodations and honoring your needs gives you opportunity to trust yourself. Forcing yourself past thresholds of capacities is similar to winding a spring beyond its capacity to maintain stability. Fluctuations beyond thresholds are typified as movements of anger to rage. Rage is a breaking of stability.

Increasing thresholds for emotional capacity in the body is the distinct purpose of the framework articulated in this theory. The methods described in previous sections allow for a microscopic orientation to the body. The body is where emotions are experienced. If there are repressed emotions in the body, there is an upper limit on emotions that can be processed in real time. Removing those upper limits only happens through the psychosomatic processes as described herein, or processes similar to them.

The premise of this theory bears repeating. Emotions are a ***body-based mechanism***. Thoughts influence emotions. But, processing emotional energy *as a human* happens **only** through the vehicle of the physical body. Reaching equanimity is **not** a mental exercise, it is an emotional one. Equanimity is a natural result of

Body Integration

integrating the body. Integrating the body is a process of synergizing the mind, the emotions, and the body.

Unresolved past emotional stagnancy **is** the upper limit on your emotional capacity. You cannot move beyond that capacity until you face that stagnancy locked in your body. As theorized herein, chronic pain (pain of an area lasting longer than 3 months) is an indicator of unresolved trauma. There is no one who can make the decision to face this trauma other than the one who is experiencing it.

There is no savior coming to wipe it all away in this sense. Noticing where you are unwilling to address conflict in your life allows you to take on the role of directing your life. If you find yourself with an unwilling to resolve conflict, it will result as tension in your body. Being able to fully receive process your experience in present-time requires resolution of your past that is held as tension. In doing so, you can embrace the perfect symmetry of this moment.

Being free to generate emotions, of any type, in the present is a result of doing the work necessary to embrace the symmetry of existing. From this symmetry, a distinct choice to resonate in joy, happiness, or any number of other emotions is possible. Consciously generating emotions in real time is reserved only for those who are willing to address any obstacle in the way of this immense power. Justifications for accepting anything less than perfect symmetry are many. The reason to disobey these justifications and proceed beyond those fallacies is singular – your freedom.

Section 7: Paradigm of Integrity

Integration, in this context, implies that it occurs as a way of life. It's axiomatic that *movement* of a living body is always happening. There is never a moment where symmetry is not possible.

Body Integration

In this way, the *practice* of integrating the body is **not** something that should ever be put on a "to do" list. That is missing the point entirely. Moments of integration happen in every moment you remember that you can become more aware of your experience. Maybe you train yourself to remember this as you first see sunlight in the morning, or as you turn on your phone, or computer. Perhaps remembering involves posting sticky notes all over your reality to remind yourself. Maybe you get a tattoo that reminds you. Maybe you set an alarm clock every hour. The method of remembering to become ever-more aware of your experience is limited only by your imagination. *That you remember* and **do** is what matters. Knocking it off your to-do list first thing in the morning or waiting till the evening to "get it done" is not the paradigm entailed herein. There is never not a moment to be more deliberate in the thoughts you use, the emotions you generate, and the movements you make.

Increasing the quality of experience as a base value *is the imperative* in this way of life. Facing the pain (whether its mental anguish, emotional turmoil, physical discomfort, or any combination thereof) with proper attention on what the body requires to release the tension/anguish/turmoil is primary. Supplemental to that is being responsive to the integrative approach of the mind-body connection. This begins to align a type of movement throughout the day that is prioritized to take actions toward health more consistently during the day.

Section 8: Eliminating Waste

As a recurring daily event where there exists opportunity to bring into symmetry the integrity of your body, eliminating waste is a prime method to experiment. In this context, eliminating waste occurs through urinating, defecating, coughing, sneezing, farting, burping, or any combination thereof.

Body Integration

There is no pre-defined sequence to practice here. There is only using the methodologies outlined herein to practice in becoming more skilled at eliminating the waste out of your body in proper manner.

As you generate more cognizance in this process, it can act as a metaphor for how you eliminate out of your experience that which does not support you any longer.

Your approach to both is a feedback loop into each. Keeping things in your life longer than what they can be useful is unhealthy. If you fail to eliminate the waste of your body, you will get sick. Eliminating it with grace gives you a newfound sense of integrity.

These decisions are ones you already make daily. Will you make them with increasing awareness and skill, or continue in the assumption that you need not improve your purification rituals?

Section 9: Additional One Minute Workouts

The following patterns assumes a practiced degree of proficiency with the Core Focus Sequence as previously discussed in this book. To reiterate, that is 1) coccygeus, 2) perineum, 3) abdominals, 4) back extensors, and 5) the obliques. What follows are supplemental patterns to that core pattern. In describing the following patterns, the word "core" refers to this base pattern. Perform each of these patterns for at least one minute in length. The goal is to incrementally increase the length of time per session.

Note: if you suffer from any pelvic floor issues, such as hemorrhoids, vaginal prolapse, or any other such condition, it may be advisable to consult a Physical Therapist before beginning any such exercises. Additionally, depending on your current state, it may require you to work toward being able to do inversions as a preliminary step, then engage the breathing patterns below. If

Body Integration

you're unsure, a safe measure to test this is to lay on the ground, bring your heels in toward your buttocks to a comfortable position, and raise your hips off the ground till your back and femurs are in a generally straight line. Then begin the core pattern engaging the muscles to no more than 10% contraction. This is a simple, safe form of inversion.

Additionally, if you suffer from any other condition that prevents you from finding a position laying on the floor, such as if you have a partially severed spinal cord and have limited mobility in your arms and legs, these patterns can be modified to your needs. You will need to adopt mental flexibility to take the goal of the pattern and adapt it to your situation.

9.1 Seated Gluteus Wave

In any comfortable sitting position, engage the core to 30% contraction output. Take a full breath in and allow for a comfortable slow exhale while engaging contraction in the left gluteus maximus. Engage to 75% contraction to a distinct sense of contraction is felt in the gluteus mediums. It's okay if there is a sense of contraction in the quadriceps and hamstrings. As the exhale reaches its valley, relax all muscle contractions except for the core, keep it at 30%. Take another full breath in, begin comfortable slow exhale while engaging the right gluteus muscles in similar manner. Allow the exhale to reach its valley. Continue with this back-and-forth waving contraction from left to right, exploring the somatic edge of muscular contraction. Where does the contraction bring a new sense of proprioceptive awareness in the muscle? Explore these zones with gentleness. One minute should ideally last for about two full cycles of breath allowing for contraction of the left and right at least one time each.

9.2 Standing Gluteus Wave

In any comfortable standing position, engage the core to 30% contraction output. Take a full breath in and allow for a

Body Integration

comfortable slow exhale while engaging contraction in the left gluteus maximus. Engage to 75% contraction to a distinct sense of contraction is felt in the gluteus mediums. It's okay if there is a sense of contraction in the quadriceps and hamstrings. As the exhale reaches its valley, relax all muscle contractions except for the core, keep it at 30%. Take another full breath in, begin comfortable slow exhale while engaging the right gluteus muscles in similar manner. Allow the exhale to reach its valley. Continue with this back-and-forth waving contraction from left to right, exploring the somatic edge of muscular contraction. Where does the contraction bring a new sense of proprioceptive awareness in the muscle? Explore these zones with gentleness. One minute should ideally last for about two full cycles of breath allowing for contraction of the left and right at least one time each.

9.2 For More, Go Here

For additional patterns, navigate to https://MichaelPhoenix.Me/body-integration

Other Titles by Michael Phoenix

Visit https://MichaelPhoenix.me for more.

- "Of the First Magnitude" series
    - Facing Revelation: An Emerging
    - iRise: An Algorhythm of Freedom
    - Quantum Engineering: Introspecting the Rabbit Hole
    - Algorhythmic Insight: Poetic Analysis of the Journey

www.ingramcontent.com/pod-product-compliance
Lightning Source LLC
Chambersburg PA
CBHW031501040426
42444CB00007B/1163